Anger
Management
Skills

Workbook for Kids

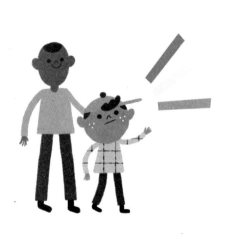

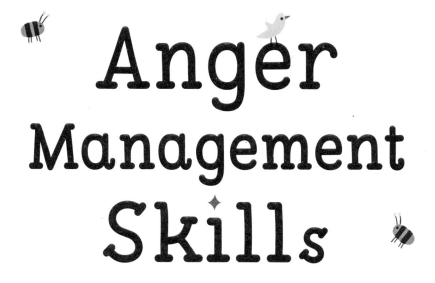

Anger Management Skills

Workbook for Kids

40 Awesome Activities to Help Children Calm Down, Cope, and Regain Control

Amanda Robinson

Z KIDS • NEW YORK

Text copyright © 2020 by Penguin Random House LLC

Illustration copyright © 2020 by Pau Morgan

All rights reserved.

Published in the United States by Z Kids, an imprint of Zeitgeist, a division of Penguin Random House LLC, New York.

penguinrandomhouse.com

Zeitgeist is a trademark of Penguin Random House LLC

ISBN: 9780593196601

Book design by Aimee Fleck

Printed in the United States of America

5 7 9 10 8 6 4

First Edition

Dedicated to my parents

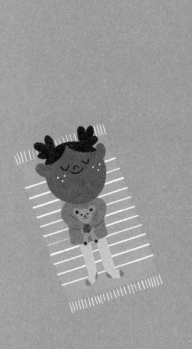

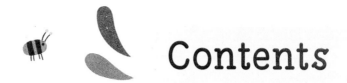

Contents

Chapter Three: **Learn Self-Control**

Chapter Four: **Talk Back to Your Triggers**

Chapter Five: **Solve Problems**

Chapter Six: **Speak Up!**

Chapter Seven: **Feel Great!**

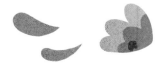

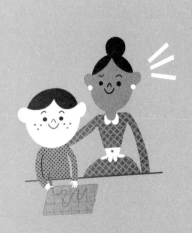

Introduction for Parents

Welcome to *Anger Management Skills Workbook for Kids*. I'm Amanda Robinson, a licensed professional counselor and registered play therapist. Right now, you might be feeling that your child is the only one with challenges. But your child has company. I have been working with children in therapy since 2013, and in that time, I have seen plenty of them struggle to regulate their emotions. Some kids already possess the skills needed to control their anger, but others lack the tools they need to express it in healthy and effective ways. (Truthfully, sometimes adults have trouble with this, too!)

Parents (I use *parents* for simplicity here, but I'm also referring to caregivers and guardians) play the most important role in helping their children feel and behave better. You are truly the experts of your own children, and you can be just as effective as therapists if you have the right tools and knowledge. That's why, for best results, you should work on this book together with your child. You'll know what skills are being taught, and can remind your child to use them.

In using this book, you will see improvement in your child's behavior, both at home and at school. You'll start to feel more connected to them, and they'll get along better with their siblings. You may even find the tools of this book useful for yourself! As we know, children mimic the behavior that they see, and they need the adults in their lives to model a healthy expression of anger.

Know that, just as with any skill, these tools will need to be practiced and may take some time to sink in. No book or intervention can change behavior overnight. You're probably feeling tired and out of patience at this point, but stay consistent, and you will see change with time.

At the end of every chapter, you'll find a "Keep It Going!" section with games and exercises that will give your child more practice with the anger management skills. These activities are designed for the whole family to do together. Remind family members to listen to each other with understanding, not judgment, during these activities. No one should be forced to talk if they don't want to.

Once your child has mastered the skills in this book, they (with your participation and guidance) will know how to identify their feelings, challenge negative thinking patterns, and practice healthy coping skills when angry feelings arise. Your family will feel better, and life will feel a bit more peaceful for everybody.

Note that this book is not intended to replace therapy. If your child meets any of the following criteria, you should seek professional support for anger management:

- The child's anger problems are new and follow a traumatic event.

- The behavior is causing the child serious trouble at school.

- The behavior is interfering with the child's ability to socialize with other kids, and the child is often excluded from playdates.

- The child's self-esteem is suffering.

- The child is showing other signs that they're struggling—for example, difficulty sleeping, lack of interest in activities they usually enjoy, frequent headaches or stomachaches, and so on.

- The child has directly asked to talk to someone outside the family.

Introduction for Kids

Hello! I'm Amanda and I wrote this book to help you learn about your anger and how you can control it. Did you know that it's normal for humans to have anger? It's not a bad thing at all! But sometimes when we're mad, we do things that aren't helpful, like slamming doors or hitting someone. These actions can hurt others, and they get us into trouble. If that has happened to you, you're not alone. Lots of kids (and even some adults) don't know how to control their anger and need help.

This is where this book comes in! It's full of fun activities that are written for kids your age. It's best to do them with an adult so you can both learn about where your anger comes from and what you can do to "get it out."

Learning these skills will take practice and time, just like when you learned how to hold a pencil or ride a bike. Once you've got them down, you'll feel calmer and more in control. You might also find that you get in trouble less often, and get along better with family and friends.

Let's get started on your journey through the book! I will be with you every step of the way.

Chapter One

Say Hello— and Goodbye— to Your Anger

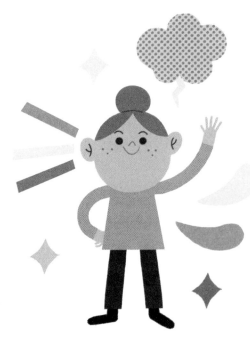

This workbook will teach you tools for coping with your anger in healthy and helpful ways, but you can't learn to control your anger until you understand where it comes from! The activities in this chapter will give you the words to label anger and similar feelings. You will also learn to recognize what factors (both inside and outside your mind) set off your anger, and how your actions affect those around you. At the end of this (and every) chapter, you'll find fun activities you can do with your family to get some extra practice with these skills. And at the end of the book, you'll find an answer key in case you need a little help or want to check your answers.

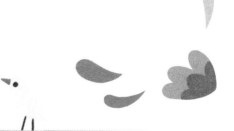

Decode Angry Feelings

Have you noticed that feelings come in different levels? Some moments, you might only feel a little bit cranky, while other times you might feel much more upset. You might also find that your feelings can change quickly from weak to strong. Below, you'll find several words for anger, but they're all written in a number code! Use the key to the right to help you figure out what the words are.

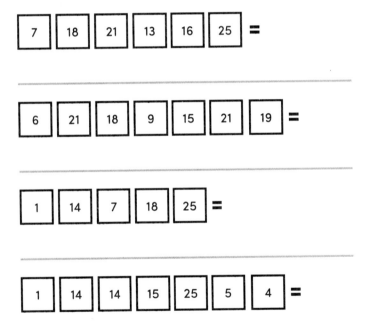

| 7 | 18 | 21 | 13 | 16 | 25 | **=** |

| 6 | 21 | 18 | 9 | 15 | 21 | 19 | **=** |

| 1 | 14 | 7 | 18 | 25 | **=** |

| 1 | 14 | 14 | 15 | 25 | 5 | 4 | **=** |

| 6 | 18 | 21 | 19 | 20 | 18 | 1 | 20 | 5 | 4 | **=** |

1 = A	14 = N
2 = B	15 = O
3 = C	16 = P
4 = D	17 = Q
5 = E	18 = R
6 = F	19 = S
7 = G	20 = T
8 = H	21 = U
9 = I	22 = V
10 = J	23 = W
11 = K	24 = X
12 = L	25 = Y
13= M	26 = Z

If anger had a temperature, which of those feelings on the previous page do you think would feel the "hottest?" Write the words on the lines next to the thermometer, listing them in order from weakest (at the bottom) to strongest (at the top).

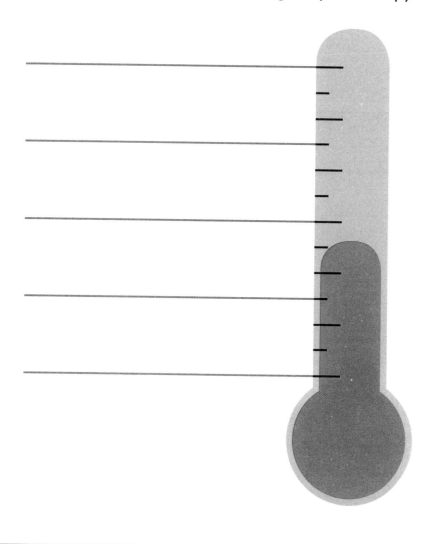

It Bugs Me When . . .

These insects are buzzing about different things that can make kids mad. Color the insects that are talking about something that annoys or angers you. If it doesn't make you feel mad, leave it blank.

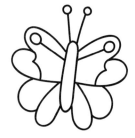

If I have to go somewhere
I don't want to go

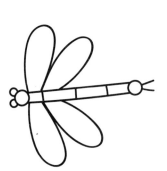

If someone borrows my stuff
without asking first

If I get yelled at

If someone teases me

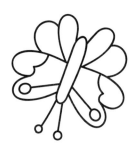

If I get in trouble

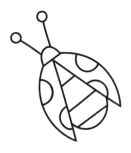

If someone hits me

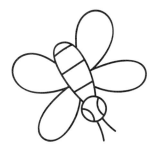

If no one seems to
care about me

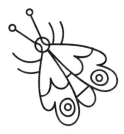

If I have to do something
I don't want to do

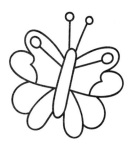

If someone keeps doing
something after I've
asked them to stop

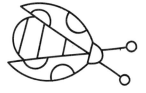

If I lose at a game

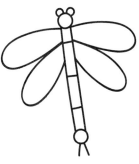

If I want something
I can't have

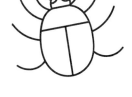

If I'm not getting the
attention I need

If I don't get to make my
own decisions

Can you think of any other things that make you feel grumpy or angry? Write them on the lines:

Anger Volcano

Activity 2 taught you about things outside our bodies and minds that can upset us. However, sometimes the things that trigger our frustration are invisible and come from our own minds. When we try to push these feelings down and ignore them, they don't go away. Instead, they build up until we explode. Anger is a lot like a volcano that way—we can't always see stuff that's boiling under the surface, but we all notice when it starts to erupt!

Color the volcano picture on the next page, and then check off the invisible thoughts and feelings listed below that set off your anger.

☐ When I don't feel listened to

☐ When my feelings are hurt

☐ When I get embarrassed

☐ When I think I'm not good at something

☐ When I'm bored

☐ When I'm scared or nervous

☐ When I feel left out

☐ When I make a mistake and feel bad

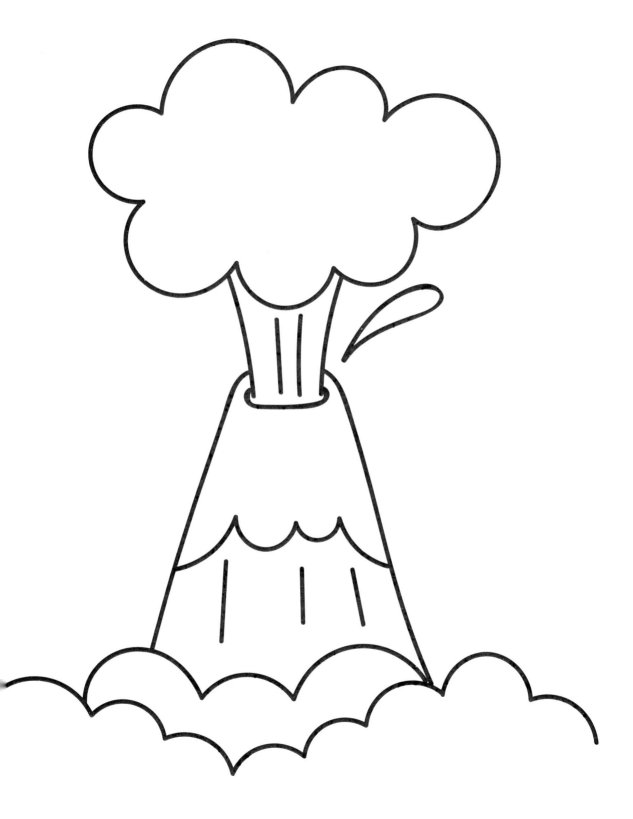

Roar! My Anger Is Like A . . .

We often show signs of our feelings in our faces and bodies. When we're happy, we may smile more, and if we're scared, we might freeze or bite our lips. We show signs of being angry, too. Below is a list of body signals that many people experience when they're angry. Circle the ones that are true about you.

Clenched fists   Hard to talk

Face gets red   Frowning

Breathing fast   Face feels hot

Heart pounding   Clenched jaw

Feel like crying   Thirsty

Hard to think clearly   Chest feels tight

Now, draw a picture of an animal that you feel and act like when you're really angry:

My anger is like a

How I Show Anger

When you feel furious about something, what do you do with that energy?

   Maybe you do or say things that hurt other people or that get you in trouble. You probably do things that you would never do when you feel calm and happy! While it's not okay to hurt people or things, it doesn't mean that you're a bad person. Everyone makes mistakes sometimes. It's important to be honest about the things you do when you're mad, so that you can learn better ways to show your feelings.

   On the next page is a short story about Ava, who gets upset and shows her anger in unhelpful ways. Read the story to yourself, or have an adult read it to you. Circle the feeling words you see, and underline actions that you've taken when you're angry.

Ava Got Angry

Ava was playing in her room when her brother came in without asking. Ava felt annoyed, because he's supposed to ask first. She yelled at him to leave her room. When he didn't go, Ava felt frustrated. She called him a mean name and hit him. She also stomped her feet and made a scary face. When her brother still didn't leave, Ava became furious. She threw her toys and pushed her brother out of the room. Then she slammed the door behind him.

Keep It Going!

1 DRAW YOUR ANGER

Each family member draws a picture about something that makes them angry. When everyone is finished drawing, reveal your pictures to one another and describe them.

SKILL BEING PRACTICED:

identifying external triggers of anger

2 MAKE A VOLCANO

This project gets messy, so do it outdoors!

1. Before starting, reread Activity 3 so that the connection between anger and volcanoes is fresh in everyone's mind.
2. Fill a 2-liter bottle almost to the top with warm water, and set it on the ground.
3. Squeeze about six drops of dish soap into the bottle.
4. Add two tablespoons of baking soda.
5. Quickly and carefully pour in ¼ cup vinegar, and then move out of the way! As the volcano erupts, everyone shouts out an internal trigger.

SKILL BEING PRACTICED:

identifying internal triggers of anger

3   CREATE ANIMAL PUPPETS

Using paper lunch sacks and art supplies, each family member creates their own animal puppet. The child who is completing the workbook creates the same animal they drew in Activity 4. Family members then use their puppets to interview each other's animal on what it feels and does when angry. Here are some interview questions to get you started:

SKILLS BEING PRACTICED:

identifying triggers, describing what anger physically feels like, and identifying unhelpful behaviors

- What kind of animal are you?
- What makes you angry?
- What do you do when you get angry?
- Where do you feel the anger in your body?

4   DRAW DIFFERENT LEVELS OF ANGER

Review the different levels of anger in Activity 1. Each family member should draw a different face to represent each feeling. How does an annoyed face look different from a frustrated or furious face?

SKILL BEING PRACTICED:

understanding intensity levels of anger

5   PLAY WAR

Play War in teams using a regular deck of cards. Anytime an ace is played, the team that put it down will name an unhelpful angry behavior. Whoever wins each round keeps the pile of cards, and whoever has the biggest pile in the end wins the game. Answers should be kept general, and not specify or criticize any one person's behavior.

SKILL BEING PRACTICED:

identifying unhelpful behaviors

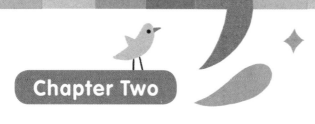

Chapter Two

Create Calm

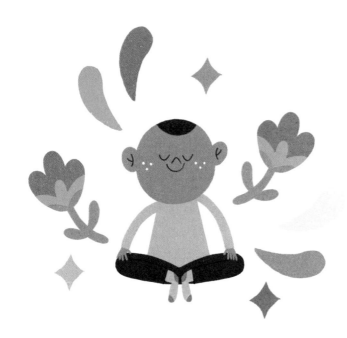

Now that you have named your anger, what triggers it, and how it feels, you can start learning some skills for coping with it. All of the ideas in this chapter will help you get calm, cool, and relaxed. It's important to know how to soothe yourself when you're trying to gain control of your emotions. You can use these exercises even when you feel fine! The more you practice them, the easier they'll be when you're upset and need them the most.

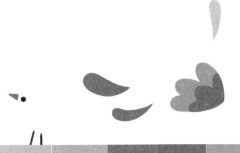

Breathe in Good Vibes

One of the best ways to get rid of stress and find calm is to practice breathing. You might think it sounds silly to practice breathing, because you can already do it without thinking about it! But breathing for relaxation is different from normal breathing. It means paying attention to how you do it, as well as how it makes you feel. Try out the breathing exercises here, and put a check in the boxes after you've completed them.

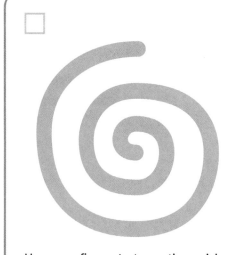

Use your finger to trace the swirl above. Breathe in when you trace from the tail into the middle, and breathe out when you trace from the middle out. See if you can make your breath last longer and longer each time!

Use your finger to trace the square below as you follow the instructions.

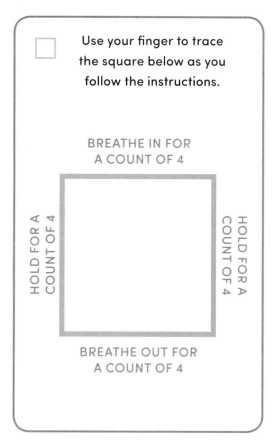

BREATHE IN FOR A COUNT OF 4

HOLD FOR A COUNT OF 4

HOLD FOR A COUNT OF 4

BREATHE OUT FOR A COUNT OF 4

Lie on your back on the floor, and put a stuffed animal on your stomach. Breathe in and out. Does the stuffed animal rise and fall as you breathe? If it does, you're doing it right! If not, keep practicing getting the air all the way down into your belly.

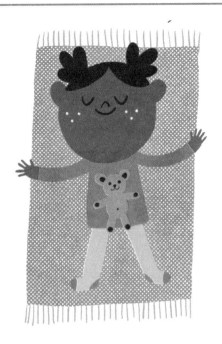

Close your eyes and pretend you're blowing out the candles on your birthday cake. Remember, you have to blow out long and steady if you want all the flames to go out in one breath!

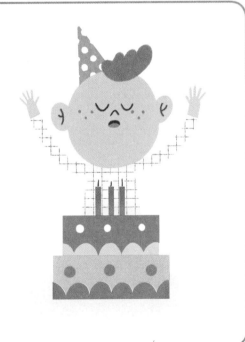

Mad Muscles

When we get stressed or frustrated, we sometimes tense our muscles without knowing we're doing it. This can leave our bodies feeling rigid. Muscle exercises will help you notice when your body is feeling tense, so you can take action to relax it.

Below are several muscle exercises, but one word is missing from each exercise. Fill in the blank with your own ideas using the clues in parentheses. Feel free to be silly with them! When you're finished filling in the blanks, give the exercises a try. Hold each muscle for 10 seconds, and then relax.

Curl your toes under like you're standing

in _____ .
(SOMETHING SQUISHY)

Squeeze your fists like you're juicing a

_____ .
(TYPE OF FRUIT)

Lift your arms up like you're reaching

for a _____ .
(SOMETHING HIGH IN THE SKY)

Bite down with your jaws like you're

trying to chew a _____ .
(SOMETHING HARD)

Bend your knees and squat like you're

going to sit on a _____ .
(PIECE OF FURNITURE)

Scrunch up your face like you have a

_____ on your nose.
(TYPE OF INSECT)

Hold in your stomach like a

_____ is sitting on you.
(HEAVY ANIMAL)

Fetch the Stretch

Stretching can do a lot of different things for you. It can help you wake up in the morning, get your muscles ready before playing sports, and relax when you're feeling flustered. Stretching can make your body feel much better, and a calmer body can lead to a calmer mind.

Here's one stretch you can try. It's called child's pose, so it's perfect for you! Try holding it for 10 seconds.

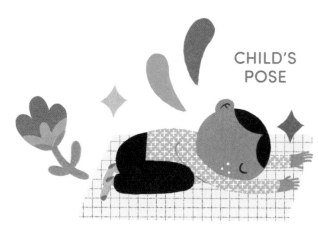

CHILD'S POSE

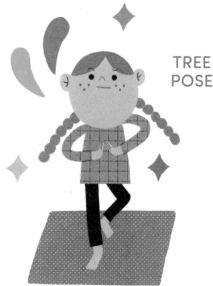

TREE POSE

Another good stretch to try is called tree pose. Make sure you try it out for 10 seconds on each foot.

Are you ready to practice these stretches more? Ask an adult to slowly read the story below. When you hear the word "tree," get into tree pose, and when you hear the word "child," get into child's pose.

In the park, a child is climbing up a tree. The tree is very tall! The child holds onto branches to climb higher and higher. The tree branches are strong, so the child feels safe. The child is wearing bright blue, so it's easy to see them in the tree.

What Is Your Calm Place?

Another way you can get calm is by meditating, which is really just a fancy way of saying that you notice what's happening in your mind and body right now. Ask an adult to slowly and quietly read you the script below, while you follow along in your mind.

Get comfy in your seat and close your eyes. Take three deep breaths, breathing out slowly each time. One . . . two . . . three. Now, think about a place where you feel relaxed and happy. It could be a place you've been before or a place you make up in your mind. Pretend that you're in that place. Notice the things you can see . . . the things you can hear . . . the things you can touch . . . the things you can smell . . . and the things you can taste. Notice how you feel in this calm place.

Now, use the space below to draw a picture of the calm place you imagined. Remember to include the things you could see, hear, touch, smell, and taste! Add as many details as you can.

In my calm place, I feel

All Aboard the Feelings Express

Choo choo! The Feelings Express has pulled into the station. Before it can leave, it needs to refuel. Write down as many positive or negative feeling words that you can think of to help it get going again. A couple of examples have been provided.

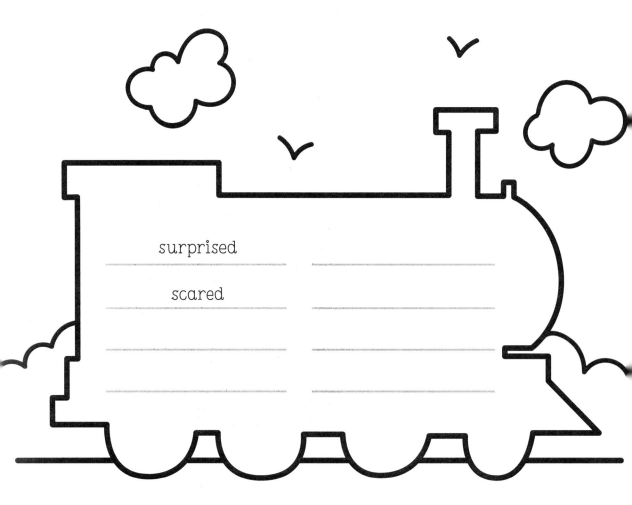

surprised

scared

There are lots of healthy ways to express your feelings to others. See if you can find all of the ideas in the word search below.

```
U  V  B  L  F  V  H  Z  B  T
B  S  Z  M  G  A  X  W  H  W
Q  H  E  P  G  E  M  D  Y  R
U  I  Q  P  A  Z  N  R  S  I
N  N  M  W  U  D  L  A  I  T
O  J  W  R  P  P  A  W  N  E
M  D  T  S  E  A  P  N  G  V
S  X  A  X  L  N  I  E  C  Y
S  W  L  V  J  N  Y  N  T  E
W  K  K  D  O  P  S  O  T  S
```

Talk   Write   Draw

Dance   Sing   Use puppets

                Paint

Gratitude, Not Attitude

Sometimes it's important to think and talk about our problems. But if we only think about our problems and never the good stuff, we won't feel very good about life! Gratitude is a feeling that means appreciating what you have. Remembering to notice the good things every day will fill you with gratitude, and the more gratitude you have, the less angry you will feel.

These boxes list lots of things that people are often grateful for:

PEOPLE

Family

Friends

Classmates

Teacher/
School staff

Doctor/Dentist

NEEDS

Food

Water

Home

Health

Safety

FUN THINGS

Toys

Books

Trips

Electronics

Hobbies

OTHER

Pets

Your talents

Your strengths

Kindness

Draw the three things that you feel most grateful for, and then label them below the picture. You might even be able to think of something that wasn't in one of the boxes!

Keep It Going!

1 MUSCLE RELAXATION

Refer back to the muscle relaxation exercises in Activity 2. With the child leading the way, the family can practice the exercises together.

SKILL BEING PRACTICED:

muscle relaxation

2 GRATITUDE AT DINNER

At dinner (or the next family meal), family members can take turns naming one thing they are grateful for. Keep this tradition up every day!

SKILL BEING PRACTICED:

gratitude

3 FAMILY STRETCHING STORY

Refer back to the yoga poses in Activity 3. Work together as a family to create another story, either using the same poses or different ones. While one person reads the story, the rest of the family will get into the poses.

SKILL BEING PRACTICED:

stretching

4 FEELINGS CHARADES

Write each feeling word below on a small piece of paper. Take turns selecting a piece of paper and acting out the feeling (using facial expressions and body movements) while the other family members try to guess what is being expressed.

SKILL BEING PRACTICED:

identifying feelings

SUGGESTIONS FOR FEELINGS:

- happy
- excited
- confused
- frustrated
- annoyed
- furious
- scared
- bored
- sad

5 BUBBLE BREATHING

Family members can take turns blowing a big bubble for a count of five. See if you can do it without making the bubble pop! Notice how the breathing technique required in blowing bubbles is the same one required in breathing for relaxation: deep inhales with steady exhales.

SKILL BEING PRACTICED:

breathing

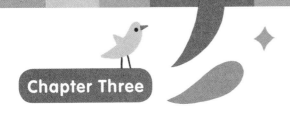

Chapter Three

Learn Self-Control

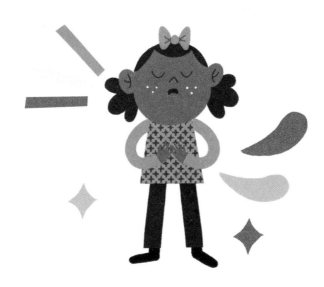

The self-calming skills you learned in the last chapter help relax your mind and body. When you're calm, you can more easily take control of your anger and other feelings. In this chapter, you'll learn how to exercise patience and think more positively about both yourself and the world. You'll also practice planning ahead and thinking about consequences, so that you can make good decisions.

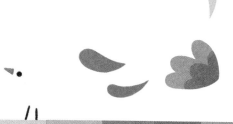

Think Things Through

Let's spend a little time learning about your brain. The middle part of your brain holds your feelings, and it likes to act quickly, without thinking. We can call this your Feeling Brain. The Feeling Brain is the one in charge when you get angry and yell or throw something without really meaning to.

THINKING BRAIN

FEELING BRAIN

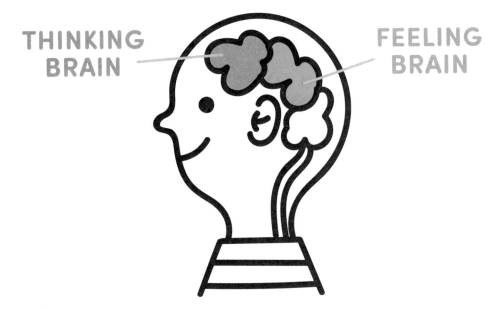

The front of your brain likes to think things through first before taking action. We can call this your Thinking Brain. It's in charge when you think calmly about a problem and come up with a smart plan. The Thinking Brain is not better than the Feeling Brain; both have important jobs. However, in order to get control of your feelings and make good choices, the Thinking Brain needs to be exercised!

Help the Thinking Brain get stronger by doing these puzzles:

RIDDLE:

It's as light as a feather, but even the strongest person can't hold it for more than five minutes. What is it?

UNSCRAMBLE THE WORDS:

BNAIR _____

NKTHI _____

LEEF _____

LACM _____

FILL IN THE BLANK:

🍎 + 🍎 + 🍎 = 9

🍎 + 🍎 + 🍎

+ 🍎 = _____

SOLVE THE PROBLEM:

Katy is two years older than Jackson. Blair is one year older than Katy. Jackson is eight years old.

How old are Katy and Blair?

Predict the Consequences

Any time you take an action, there will be a result. This is called a consequence, and it can be good or bad. If you help your mom wash the dishes, the consequence might be that she's happy and gives you a hug. If you break a rule at school, the consequence might be that you miss recess. Predicting what the consequences might be *before* we make a choice can help us make good decisions.

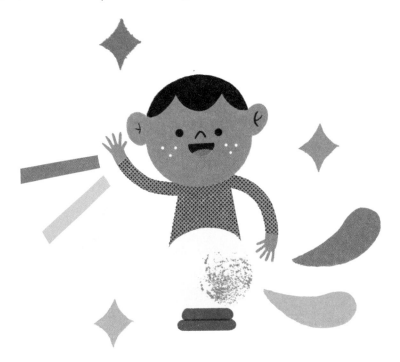

Pretend that you're a fortune-teller and can see into the future. Look into the crystal ball and help the kids on the next page figure out what one consequence of their actions might be.

Example: Charlie's mom told him he couldn't have any more cookies. Charlie decided to eat more anyway.

What do you predict will happen next?

Charlie might get in trouble with his mom.

1. Joey messed up Anna's puzzle by accident, so Anna messed up Joey's, too.

What do you predict will happen next?

2. Kaiden hit his cousin because she was using the toy he wanted.

What do you predict will happen next?

3. Mia slammed her door because her dad asked her to clean her room.

What do you predict will happen next?

Bee Patient

When we have trouble being patient while waiting, it can make us feel restless and frustrated. This little bee is impatient to get to its hive. Can you use your patience to help guide it through the maze to get home?

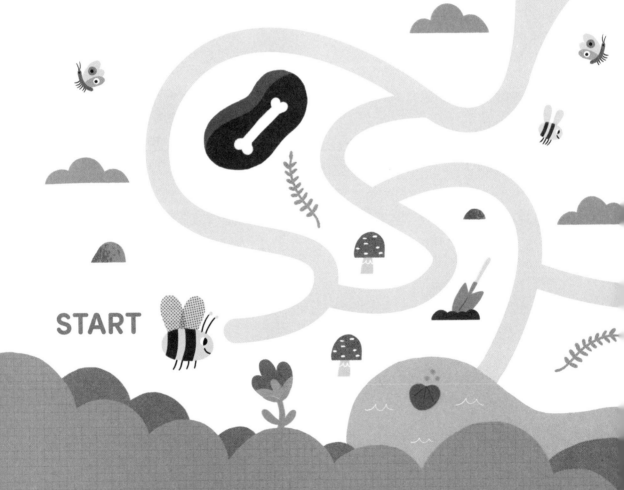

START

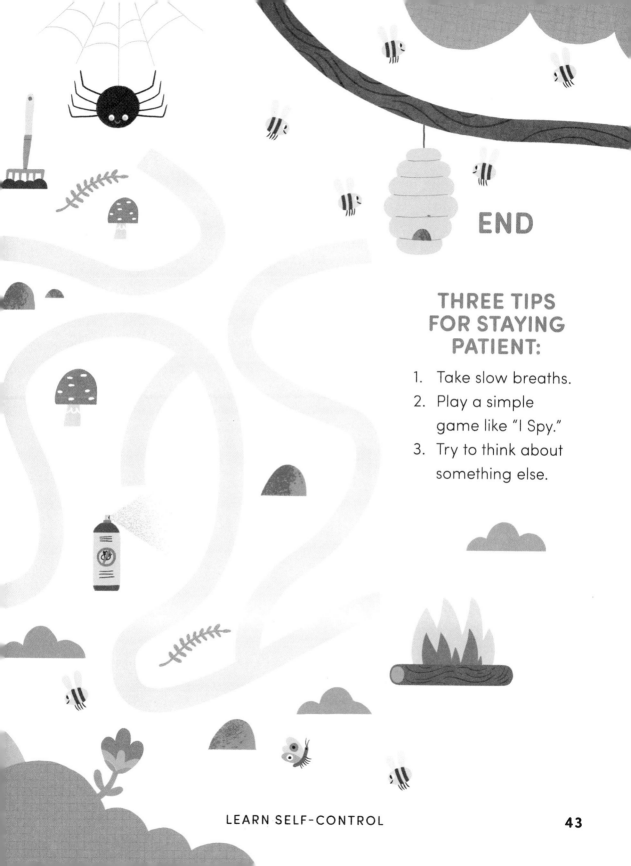

END

THREE TIPS FOR STAYING PATIENT:

1. Take slow breaths.
2. Play a simple game like "I Spy."
3. Try to think about something else.

Donut Be Hard on Yourself

After you make a mistake, it's normal to feel bad. Feeling bad or guilty is a sign that we did something wrong and need to make things right again. But we also have to remember that wrong choices don't make us bad people. There are lots of wonderful things about you. As you color each donut, say the statement under it to yourself.

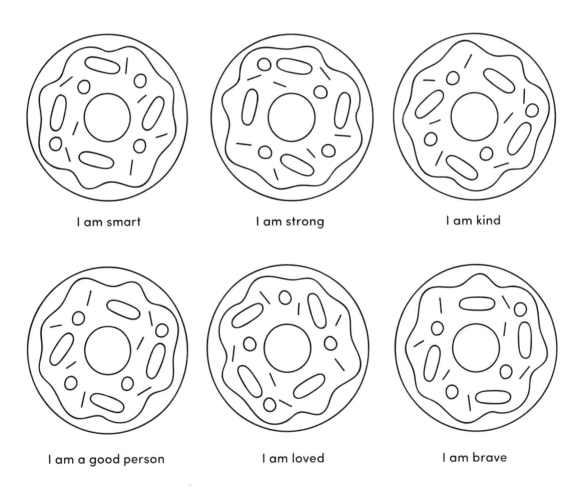

I am smart

I am strong

I am kind

I am a good person

I am loved

I am brave

Now, make a donut of your own! Color in the donut and write a positive statement below it about how to control your anger. You can copy one of the suggestions below or create your own.

SUGGESTIONS: I can do this • I can control my anger • I can stay calm

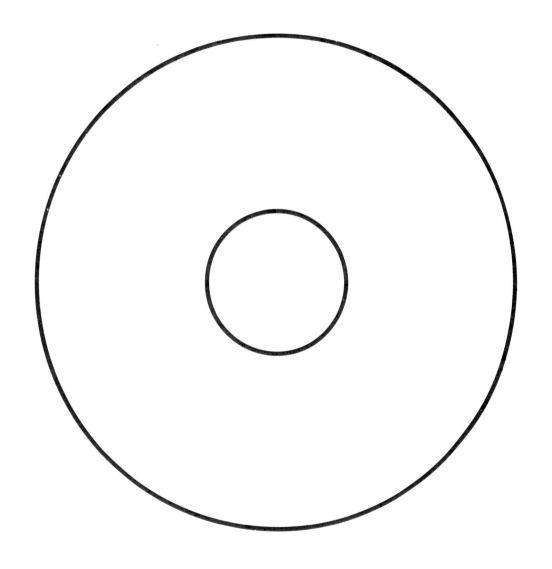

Captain Optimism

When we're in a bad mood, our thoughts can become very grumpy and focus on all the bad things, while blocking out the good things. Everyone has yucky days, and we're allowed to feel sad or cranky, but thinking too much about the bad can make us feel even worse.

That's why we have to work hard to think more positively. For this activity, pretend you're a superhero named Captain Optimism. Your job is to change all the unhelpful thoughts on the next page into more helpful ones. If you don't, negativity will take over!

Once you've completed the chart, design a superhero outfit for Captain Optimism to wear.

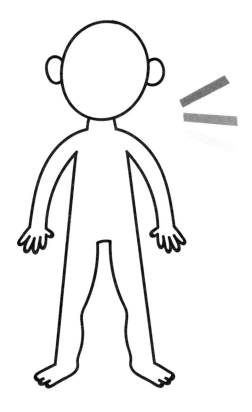

UNHELPFUL THOUGHTS	HELPFUL THOUGHTS
Example: I got a bad grade on my test. I'm not smart.	I did the best that I could. I'm smart at other things, like math.
I didn't get to play my favorite game at the arcade.	
Science is too hard for me! I can't do it.	
My parents are always too busy to play with me! It's not fair.	
My soccer team lost the game. It's all Jacob's fault.	
If Tessa doesn't sit beside me at lunch today, she's no longer my best friend.	
My grandpa made broccoli for dinner—yuck! He should've made something I like.	

Keep It Going!

1 PLAY GAMES

As a family, play fun and easy games that require patience and impulse control. Some suggestions: Red Light Green Light, the Quiet Game, and Follow the Leader.

SKILL BEING PRACTICED:

being patient

2 AFFIRMATION ART

Using art supplies, family members each write down an affirmation they most need to be reminded of, and decorate it however they like. Put your affirmation somewhere that you'll see often, such as on the refrigerator or hanging on the wall by your bed. Refer back to Activity 4 for suggestions of affirmations, if needed.

SKILL BEING PRACTICED:

positive self-talk

3 SUPERHERO FAMILY

Captain Optimism returns, this time with their trusty sidekicks! Family members create their own positive superhero names and tackle another list of negative thoughts by working together to change them into positive ones.

SKILL BEING PRACTICED:

positive thinking

- My whole day was awful because I didn't get to play outside.
- I don't want to go to Lena's birthday party. It'll be boring.

4 WOULD YOU RATHER?

Family members can play a lighthearted game of "Would You Rather?" to get everyone thinking critically. Suggestions to get started:

- Would you rather have a talking animal or be able to fly?
- Would you rather eat pizza-flavored ice cream or ice cream-flavored pizza?
- Would you rather have to swim in winter clothes or play in the snow in a swimsuit?

SKILL BEING PRACTICED:

thinking things through

5 MAKING CONNECTIONS

Each family member shares a time that they did something out of anger and experienced a negative consequence. Everyone can either write their answers down or share them out loud. Remember to listen to each other with understanding!

SKILL BEING PRACTICED:

predicting consequences

EXAMPLE:

- When I was angry, I said mean things, and it hurt Dad's feelings.

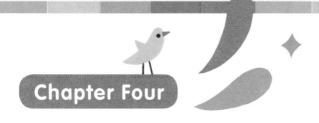

Chapter Four

Talk Back to Your Triggers

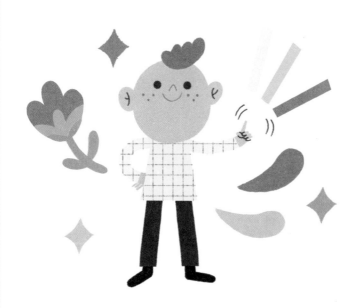

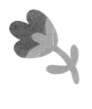

You now know how to get calm, and how to think things through. These skills can help you feel less angry and make better choices. But you're still going to get mad about stuff sometimes! You're human, and that's normal. This chapter will help you learn safe ways to get your frustration out without hurting others or getting into trouble. It may be tough at first to remember these skills when you get angry, so make sure you get lots of practice with them.

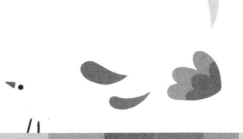

Distract Before You React

Let's say something annoying is happening. Maybe a classmate at school keeps bugging you, or you're tired of having to wait in a long line. You can feel yourself getting unhappy about it, but because you've gotten so good at managing your anger, you know you need to act now before it gets worse. Distractions can help with that!

Here are some ideas for distracting yourself:

CONSIDER YOUR SENSES

What do you currently . . .

See: _____

Hear: _____

Feel: _____

Smell: _____

Taste: _____

COUNTING

Start at 100, and count backward for as long as you can.

What number did you reach?

_____

Try to beat your record each time you practice this!

LETTER GAME

Pick a letter of the alphabet and try to think of as many words as you can that start with that letter.

List some here:

_____

_____

_____

_____

_____

DRAW

Use your opposite hand to draw a little picture. (If you're right-handed, use your left hand, and vice versa.) This requires focus!

Here are some other quick ideas for distracting yourself. Circle the ones you like:

Read a book

Make a pillow fort

Play with your pet

Play a game

Color or draw

Go outside

Put on the Brakes

Sometimes when we get angry, we want to deal with the problem right away. This isn't always possible, or a good idea. Focusing on a strong emotion can make it grow even bigger, and then it gets out of control. This is when we make choices that can get us into trouble. Sometimes it's best to stop and try to calm down before dealing with some-thing, at least until your level of anger has had a chance to go down. (Remember the anger scale in Chapter One!)

Each car contains an idea for "putting on the brakes" and calming down. As you color each car, think about the idea. Put a star next to the three ideas that you like the most.

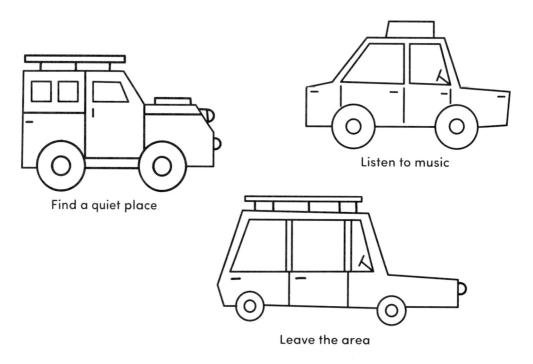

Find a quiet place

Listen to music

Leave the area

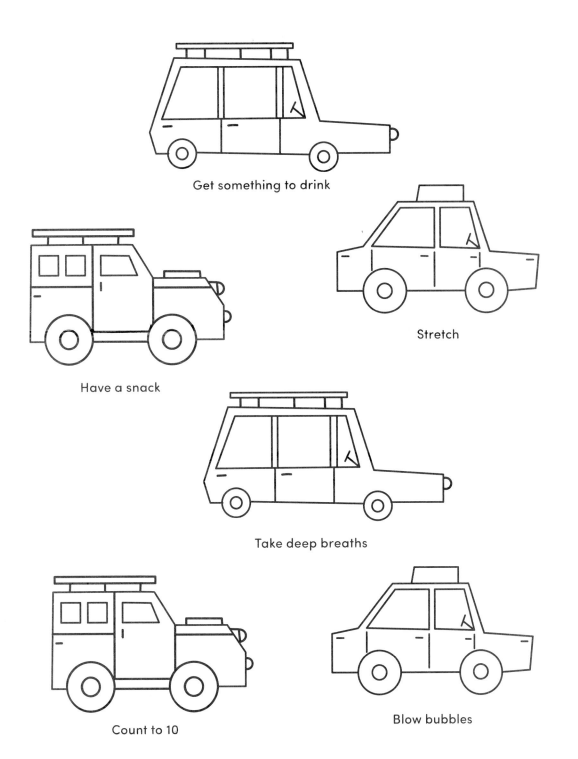

Get something to drink

Stretch

Have a snack

Take deep breaths

Count to 10

Blow bubbles

Face Your Frustration

Taking breaks and using distractions are great short-term solutions, but they won't work forever. We need to face our problems and get our angry feelings out. Think of your anger as being like a balloon—the more air you add, the bigger it gets, and then what happens? It pops! Airing your anger now and then is the best way to prevent it from overwhelming you.

Below are some ideas for expressing your anger in healthy ways. Unscramble the scrambled word in each balloon and write it down.

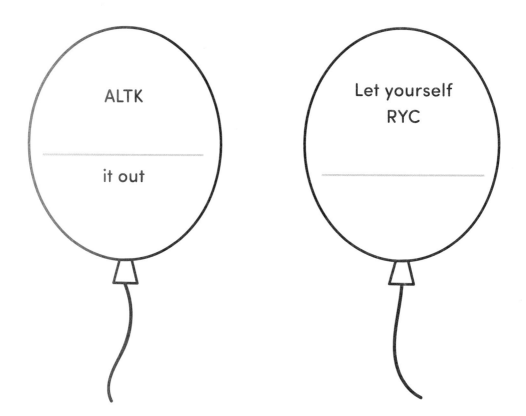

ALTK

_____

it out

Let yourself
RYC

_____

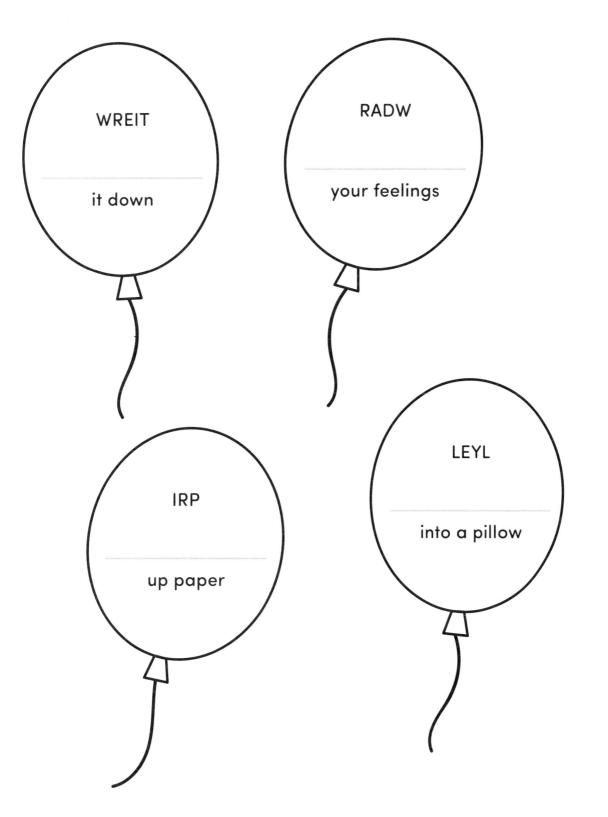

WREIT

it down

RADW

your feelings

IRP

up paper

LEYL

into a pillow

Get Moving

Anger builds up big energy in your body, and that energy can feel uncomfortable. What is one of the best ways for getting that energy out? Complete the color-by-number on the next page to find out.

1 = RED	5 = PURPLE	10 = PINK
2 = YELLOW	6 = ORANGE	11 = BROWN
3 = LIGHT GREEN	7 = LIGHT BLUE	12 = DARK GREEN
4 = DARK BLUE	8 = BLACK	BLANK SPACES = WHITE
	9 = GRAY	

Here are some physical ideas for releasing angry energy. Circle the ones you'd like to try.

Throw or hit a ball outside

Run around the yard

Break sticks

Go on a bike ride

Hit your bed with a pillow

Squeeze playdough

Do jumping jacks

Kick a ball outside

1				1	2	2	2	3		3	4	4	4	
1	1		1	1	2		2	3		3	4			
1		1		1	2		2	3		3	4	4	4	
1		1		1	2		2	3		3	4			
1		1		1	2		2	3		3	4			
1		1		1	2	2	2		3		4	4	4	
5				5	6	6	6	7		7	8	8	8	
	5		5		6		6	7		7	8		8	
		5			6		6	7		7	8	8	8	
		5			6		6	7		7	8	8		
		5			6		6	7		7	8		8	
		5			6	6	6	7	7	7	8			8
9	9	9	10	10	10		11	11		12				12
9		9	10		10		11		11	12		12		
9	9	9	10		10		11		11			12		
9	9	9	10		10		11		11			12		
9		9	10		10		11		11			12		
9	9	9	10	10	10		11	11				12		

Let It Go

Some problems need to be solved, and you'll learn all about that in the next chapter. But some issues bother us for a little while, and eventually go away. There's not much we can do about those problems, so they should be let go.

How do you know if a problem should be let go?
Ask yourself these questions:

Is the problem something that can be changed?	If the problem involves a person, did they wrong you on purpose?	Is the problem worth being upset about?

Let's practice this. Circle Yes or No to answer the questions.

Example: Your coach cancels the soccer game because of rainy weather.

Is the problem something that can be changed?	YES	NO
If the problem involves a person, did they wrong you on purpose?	YES	NO
Is the problem worth being upset about?	YES	NO

Now write down a problem that annoys
you, but can possibly be let go:

_____

Answer these questions about your problem:

Is the problem something that can be changed?	YES	NO
If the problem involves a person, did they wrong you on purpose?	YES	NO
Is the problem worth being upset about?	YES	NO

If you answer "No" to two or more of the questions, you
should try to let the problem go! To help you with that, have a
grown-up slowly and quietly read you the visualization below.

Close your eyes and take a deep breath. Let it out. Think about a problem that you're trying to let go of. Now, pretend you have a paper airplane in front of you. Picture yourself putting that problem on the paper airplane. Even though your problem may feel big, the paper plane can easily hold it. Take a deep breath in, and when you breathe out, throw your paper plane into the air. When you do, imagine a gust of wind catching hold of the plane. The plane, which still holds your problem, is so light that it soars through the air, guided by the breeze. You watch it fly farther and farther away from you. Without your problem, you feel much more at peace.

Keep It Going!

1 BALLOON VOLLEYBALL

Refer back to Activity 3, and remember how anger can be compared to filling up a balloon. With this in mind, blow up a balloon and play balloon volleyball with your family. A net isn't necessary; just work together to keep the balloon in the air. Don't let it touch the ground! When you're feeling angry, balloon volleyball is a safe way to release some of that energy.

SKILLS BEING PRACTICED:

facing frustration and moving

2 PAPER AIRPLANES

Each family member folds their own paper airplane and writes one problem or irritation on it that they want to let go of. An adult then rereads the visualization in Activity 5. Afterward, everyone throws their paper airplanes at the same time to see whose plane flies the farthest.

SKILLS BEING PRACTICED:

letting go and moving

3 HOMEMADE PLAYDOUGH

Make the recipe for homemade playdough on the next page, and have fun squishing it together to get out frustration!

SKILL BEING PRACTICED:

facing frustration

RECIPE: Mix together 1 cup flour and ¼ cup salt in a large bowl. Mix ½ cup of warm water with a few drops of food coloring in a smaller bowl. Slowly pour the water into the flour mixture, stirring as you pour. Stir until combined, and then knead until the flour is fully absorbed. If the dough is too sticky, add more flour. Store it in an airtight container.

4 FREEZE DANCE

Encourage the family to dance to high-energy music. One family member acts as the DJ, and pauses the music whenever they like. When the music stops, the dancers must freeze in place.

SKILLS BEING PRACTICED:

taking a break and moving

5 ALPHABET GAME

Take turns going through the alphabet and identifying an animal that begins with each letter (A= Alligator, B= Bear, and so on). The game will continue in order until Z has been named. Note that while playing the game, the player's mind is focused on the game and not on other problems.

SKILL BEING PRACTICED:

distraction

OTHER OPTIONAL CATEGORIES:

- food
- people's names
- cities
- household items

Chapter Five

Solve Problems

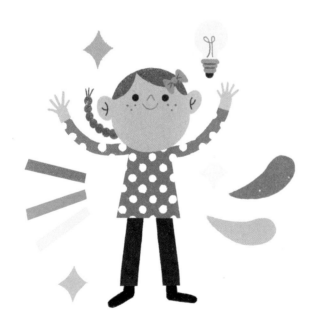

Chapter Four taught you about letting go of problems that aren't worth being upset about, or that can't be solved. However, some problems *can* be solved, and really need to be! This is one of the most important skills you'll learn in managing your anger. After all, if an issue can be calmly talked about and possibly prevented from happening, you may be able to avoid getting upset in the first place. This chapter might seem difficult at times, but it will also be the most rewarding. Once you've learned these skills, you'll feel more in charge of your feelings and challenges.

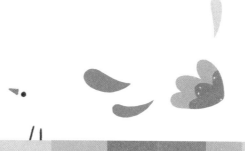

Brainstorming

Brainstorming is a funny-sounding word that means coming up with lots of ideas for something. Right now, you'll get some fun practice brainstorming so that you'll be a pro at it when you need the skill later in the chapter. In order to brainstorm, sit in a quiet place, think about the question, and say or write down whatever comes to mind. With brainstorming, no idea is too silly!

BRAINSTORMING PRACTICE 1

Name as many desserts as you can that contain chocolate:

BRAINSTORMING PRACTICE 2

Name as many words as you can that rhyme with blue:

_____   _____

_____   _____

_____   _____

_____   _____

_____   _____

BRAINSTORMING PRACTICE 3

Name as many ways as you can
to use a fork, aside from eating:

_____   _____

_____   _____

_____   _____

_____   _____

Keep Your Eyes on Compromise

When you and someone else are fighting about something, it can make you both feel mad. You probably want to win and get your own way, and you may forget that the other person has feelings, too. So what do you do? A peaceful way to fix the problem is to compromise. Here are the three steps for doing that:

1. Listen to the other person's side.

2. Share your side.

3. Brainstorm solutions and pick one together.

The people in the stories on the next page are having trouble compromising. Listen to both sides and circle the idea that you think would be fair for *both* people.

Aiden and Hannah are fighting over a toy. Aiden thinks he should get the toy first, but Hannah thinks she should. What would be a fair compromise?

A. Aiden should have the toy first because he's older and bigger.

B. They should flip a coin to see who gets to play first. After 10 minutes, they can switch.

Julie and Kim each want a cookie, but there's only one cookie left. What would be a fair compromise?

A. They should split the cookie and each take a half.

B. Whoever gets to the cookie first should get it.

Ryan is visiting his friend Ethan's house, and they can't agree on what movie to watch. What would be a fair compromise?

A. Ethan should get to pick because it's his house.

B. They should try to find a movie they can both agree on.

Learn to Empathize

Is it important to you that other people understand how you feel? If so, that's normal! All of us want to feel understood. But that also means that other people really want us to understand *them*, too. It's not always easy to know what others are feeling, but practice will help. Read the sentences below, and match them with the feeling that you think each person would be experiencing.

Feelings Words:

Haylee's dad dropped a glass, and it made a very loud sound.

Annoyed

Toby's goldfish died.

Excited

Libby found out she made the basketball team.

Sad

Emmett's little sister accidentally stepped on his foot.

Furious

Olivia's brother destroyed the painting she'd been working on for a long time.

Scared

What can we do in order to figure out what someone else is feeling? Use the key on the right to decode the answers.

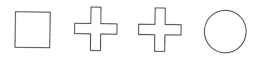

(What are their face and body doing?
Are they crying or making a mad face?)

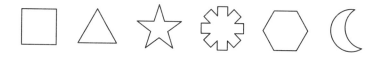

(What are they saying? Are they talking
calmly, or do they sound upset?)

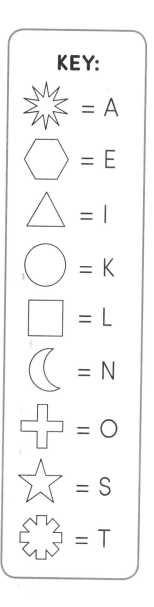

(Are they hurt or angry?)

Reframe the Problem

Your attitude is affected by the way you think about things. It's okay to feel annoyed when something bugs you, but blaming stuff on other people (even if you don't say it out loud) won't make you feel better. To help your attitude, you can try reframing. Reframing means changing the way you look at something. It won't make your angry feeling disappear completely, but it might make you feel a lot calmer.

On the next page, you'll see pairs of sentences—one will sound negative, and one will be reframed into a more positive version. Draw a red frame around the one that sounds negative and a blue frame around the one that sounds positive. Here's an example:

> My older brother beat me at a game! I hate it when he wins.

> It's nice that he wanted to play with me.

Mom cares about me and wants me to be safe.

Mom is always telling me what to do.

. . . .

I didn't make the basketball team. It's not fair.

Now I'll have more time to play with friends.

. . . .

My little sister copies everything I do! It bugs me.

She looks up to me and wants to be like me.

. . . .

My teacher wants to help me understand things better.

My teacher is making me stay after school for tutoring. I don't want to!

. . . .

My friend knocked over my Lego set. I can rebuild it in an even better way. Accidents happen.

I shouldn't have let him near it. It's all his fault.

Who Can You Count On?

When you're trying to solve a problem, it can help to talk it over with an adult you trust. Often, simply sharing your feelings with someone else can help you feel less mad. The other person may also be able to suggest solutions you hadn't thought of yourself! List people who you can rely on to help you, and draw a picture of them in the frames.

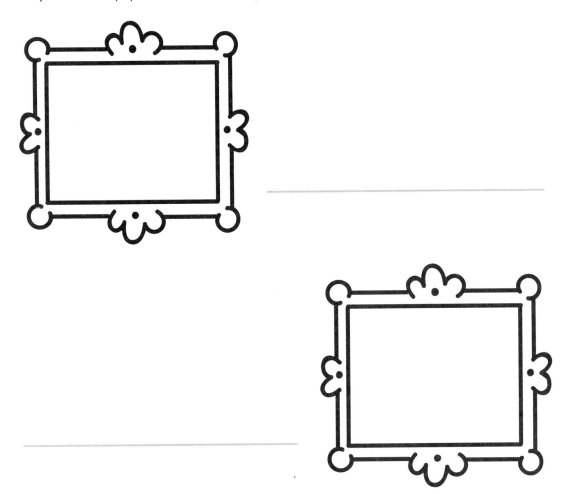

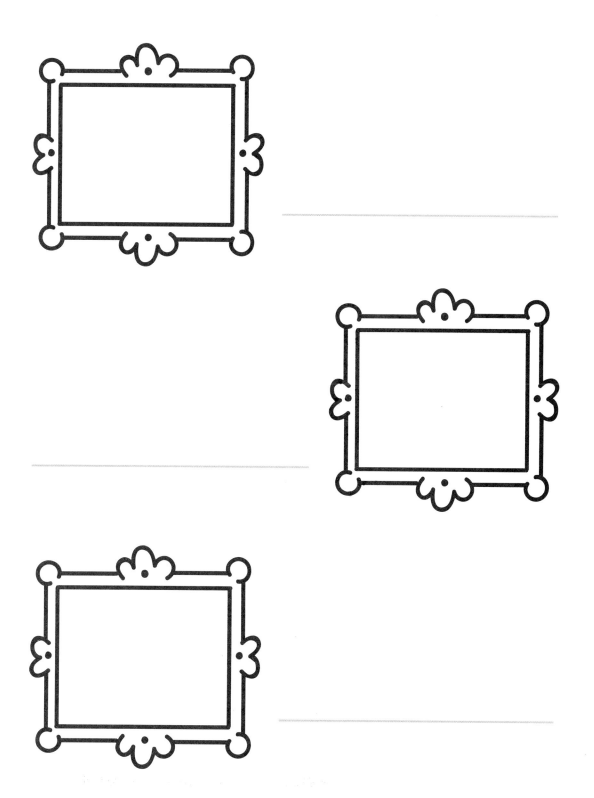

Find a Solution

All of the other activities in this chapter have led up to this moment: it's time to try solving a problem of your own! The Answer Key at the back of this book has an example of each step if you need ideas.

STEP 1 Write down a problem you've been having—something that makes you angry. (Refer back to Chapter 1, Activity 2 if you need ideas.)

_____

STEP 2 Use your new brainstorming skills to come up with some ideas for solutions. List as many as you can! For this step, don't worry about how realistic the ideas are.

_____

_____

_____

_____

STEP 3 Remember to consider the consequences of your actions! Go back to your brainstorming list in Step 2 and cross out any ideas that could:

- Hurt yourself or others
- Hurt property
- Get you in trouble

STEP 4 Show the remaining ideas to an adult. Let them help you cross off any other ideas that might not be realistic or helpful. Be open to their suggestions for solutions, too.

STEP 5 Decide on a solution to try! Remember, it's okay if the first solution you try doesn't work out. You can always return to your list and try a different one. Write down the solution you want to try first:

Keep It Going!

1 BRAINSTORM FAMILY FUN

Brainstorm fun (and free!) ways that the family can spend time together.

SKILL BEING PRACTICED:

brainstorming

2 RANDOM ACTS OF KINDNESS

Perform a random act of kindness together as a family. Adults should lead a discussion on how it would feel to be a recipient of such kindness. Ideas: pick up litter at the park, bake cookies for the elderly, leave one-dollar bills in books at the library, pay for someone else's meal at a restaurant, volunteer at an animal shelter, leave kind notes on strangers' cars.

SKILL BEING PRACTICED:

empathy

3 FAMILY MEETINGS

Once a week, hold a family meeting where household problems can be addressed and solved together. Begin and end the meeting by identifying things you appreciate about each other.

SKILLS BEING PRACTICED:

problem-solving, compromise, and empathy

4 FAMILY SKIT

Put on a skit as a family, with the child completing the workbook in charge. The skit can be on any subject and doesn't have to be related to anger— the activity itself will require skills learned from this chapter.

SKILLS BEING PRACTICED:
brainstorming, compromise, and problem-solving

5 FAMILY DANCE

Play songs about relying on others, and sing and dance to them together.

SKILL BEING PRACTICED:
counting on others

SONG SUGGESTIONS TO GET YOU STARTED:

- *Lean on Me*—Bill Withers
- *Count on Me*—Bruno Mars
- *One Call Away*—Charlie Puth
- *I Won't Let Go*—Rascal Flatts
- *Song for a Friend*—Jason Mraz
- *Ain't No Mountain High Enough*—Marvin Gaye & Tammy Terrell

Speak Up!

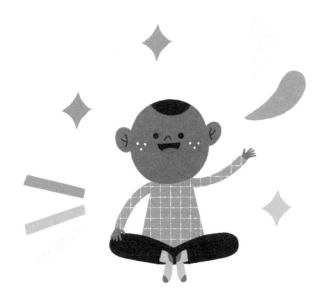

Chapter Six will help you develop and practice communication skills so that you can talk to people about how you're feeling, and also listen to their side. Mistakes will still happen now and then, so you'll also learn how to apologize and make things better with loved ones after hurting them. Knowing these skills will make it easier for you to get along with friends and family, and will be a part of your toolbox for managing anger.

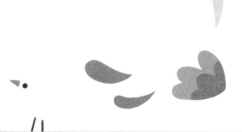

Share Your Feelings

Talking about your feelings is very important, but it's not always the easiest thing to do. You may not know exactly what you're feeling, or which words to use to describe your feelings. This activity will help you practice naming different feeling words, and remember what they mean and how they feel inside you. Use the faces below as clues to help you fill in the crossword puzzle on the next page. Each clue shows you the first letter of the word and how many letters the word has.

ACROSS

2. C _ _ _ _ _ _ _

4. H _ _ _ _

7. E _ _ _ _ _ _

8. A _ _ _ _ _ _

DOWN

1. W _ _ _ _ _ _

3. S _ _ _ _ _ _ _ _

5. S _ _ _ _ _

6. A _ _ _ _

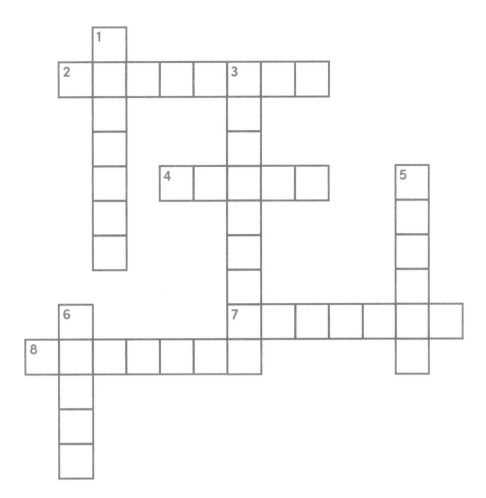

Now that your brain has had a refresher on different feeling words, it's time to practice talking about them! Tell a family member about a time when you experienced each of the feelings below. If you get stumped, ask your family member for ideas—they may be able to remember a time that you've forgotten! After you've talked about the feeling, check off the box.

☐ Angry   ☐ Surprised   ☐ Excited

☐ Scared   ☐ Annoyed   ☐ Confused

☐ Happy   ☐ Worried

"I" Messages

When you're feeling bothered by something, it's a good idea to think about what you need in order to feel better. Sometimes, you can meet your own need. Other times, you may want to share your thoughts with someone you trust so they can help you. Remember, this doesn't mean that your need will be met right away, because sometimes that's not possible! Here's what you can say:

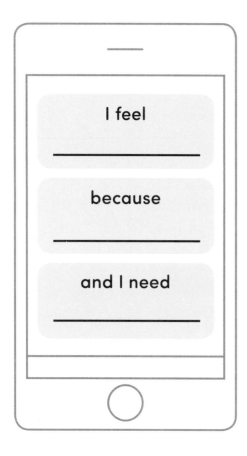

I feel

_____

because

_____

and I need

_____

EXAMPLES OF NEEDS:

- To go outdoors
  - A hug
  - Sleep or rest
    - Playtime
- Time with a parent
  - Alone time
  - Something to eat or drink
    - A break
  - A deep breath

Did you notice that the sentence in the box uses "I"? This is so you can take ownership of your feeling and need, rather than blaming it on someone else. After all, "I need alone time" sounds a lot nicer than "Get out of my room!" Practice coming up with "I" messages below. You can think of your own ideas for needs, or you can use the examples on the previous page to help you.

> Example: Your parents have been busy all day, and you've played by yourself. You're feeling bored and lonely.
>
> I feel _lonely_ because _I've played by myself all day_ and I need _time with Mom or Dad_.

1. You didn't sleep well the night before, and now you're tired.

I feel _____ because _____

and I need _____ .

2. You've been working on your homework for a long time, and you're starting to get frustrated with it.

I feel _____ because _____

and I need _____ .

3. You've had a hard day at school, and you're feeling down.

I feel _____ because _____

and I need _____ .

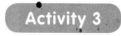

See It from the Other Side

We all see things in different ways. What might strike you as a funny joke or harmless action could upset someone else, and the opposite is also true. In order to get along well with others, we need to be able to imagine what someone else might be thinking or feeling about a situation. Some people call this "putting yourself in someone else's shoes," because you're really trying to understand how they feel. It takes some practice to see it from the other side, but once you do, you'll be able to avoid conflict more easily in the future.

Read these situations and circle the answer you think is correct. Remember to try to understand how the other person could be feeling!

Your friend Charlotte is excited to see a new movie coming out. You've already seen the movie, so you tell her the ending. Charlotte gets mad. Why?

A. She wanted to see the movie ending herself.

B. Charlotte is not nice.

Your mom just finished mopping the kitchen when you walk through with dirty shoes on. Your mom looks annoyed now. Why?

A. She's in a bad mood.

B. She worked hard to clean the floor, and now it's dirty again.

You decided to surprise your older brother by running and jumping on his back. He moves away from you and gives you an angry look. Why?

A. He's trying to be mean to you.

B. He was startled by the jump, and it might have hurt him, too.

You make a joke about your classmate's shoes, and now she looks sad. Why?

A. The joke hurt her feelings.

B. She's being a big baby.

Own Your Tone

We use our words and actions to show others how we feel, and we also use our tone of voice. It's not just what we say, but also the way we say it! When you read out loud the sentences below, try them in different tones—excited, angry, and sad. Notice how even though the words stay the same, the message changes with your tone.

READ THE SENTENCE OUT LOUD:	CHECK OFF EACH TONE YOU TRY:		
"Spaghetti is for dinner."	😄 ☐	😠 ☐	😟 ☐
"I have school today."	😄 ☐	😠 ☐	😟 ☐
"Riley is coming over to play later."	😄 ☐	😠 ☐	😟 ☐

Try saying the next few angry-sounding sentences first in a frustrated tone, and then in a calm one. This is good practice for when you're trying to work out a problem with another person. Even if you feel angry on the inside, people listen better when your tone sounds calm.

READ THE SENTENCE OUT LOUD:	CHECK OFF EACH TONE YOU TRY:			
"Put down that toy, it isn't yours."	☹	☐	☺	☐
"Stop teasing, I don't like that."	☹	☐	☺	☐
"Maddy got a cupcake, but I didn't."	☹	☐	☺	☐

Listen Up

When you're trying to solve a problem with another person, it's important that you hear their side of the issue. These three steps will help you understand why this matters, and what you can do about it.

STEP 1 How do you feel when you're not being listened to? (Circle all that apply.)

Annoyed   Angry

Hurt   Sad

Frustrated   Confused

Happy   Ignored

STEP 2 How do you think others feel when you're not listening to them? (Circle all that apply.)

Annoyed   Angry

Hurt   Sad

Frustrated   Confused

Happy   Ignored

STEP 3 Here are a few tips for listening better. Draw a small picture to illustrate each idea.

Look at the speaker	Don't interrupt
Listen to understand	Ask questions if you're unsure

Now, give these tips a try! Ask a family member to tell you about their day, and focus on looking at them, listening carefully, and not interrupting. If you're confused or have a question about something, ask.

Each time you practice this task, check off one of the boxes.

☐ ☐ ☐ ☐ ☐

Making Amends

All of us make mistakes by saying or doing things that hurt others. Apologizing can be really hard sometimes, but when we mess up, it's important that we admit it. It feels much better for *everyone* after we do! The next time you make a mistake, take these steps to make things better:

Write down the letters of the boxes with a 1 in them. Make sure you keep them in order!

| S₁ | K | R | A₁ | P | Q | Y₁ | Z | B | I₁ | O |

| M₁ | S₁ | N | S | O₁ | J | R₁ | S | D | R₁ | Y₁ |

Step 1 of making amends: _____

This time, write down the letters of the boxes with a **2** in them.

| B | G₂ | S₁ | T | A | I₂ | V₂ | W | R₁ | F | E₂ |

Row 1: B, G$_2$, S$_1$, T, A, I$_2$, V$_2$, W, R$_1$, F, E$_2$

Row 2: K$_1$, L, A$_2$, X, R$_2$, O$_1$, P, M, E$_2$, S$_1$, A$_2$

Row 3: S$_2$, Z, O$_2$, C$_1$, N$_2$, D, W$_2$, U$_1$, H$_2$, Y$_2$, S$_1$

Step 2 of making amends: _____

For the last and hardest round, write down the letters of the boxes with a **3** in them.

Row 1: D$_3$, S$_2$, A$_1$, J$_2$, O$_3$, R$_1$, S$_3$, S$_2$, B$_1$, O$_3$, C$_2$

Row 2: M$_3$, K$_1$, F$_2$, E$_3$, U$_1$, T$_1$, T$_3$, H$_3$, O$_2$, E$_1$, I$_3$

Row 3: N$_3$, L$_1$, S$_2$, G$_3$, P$_1$, K$_3$, J$_2$, I$_3$, Q$_2$, N$_3$, D$_3$

Step 3 of making amends: _____

It also helps to say what you should've done differently! Here's an example of the whole thing put together: "I'm sorry (Step 1) for knocking down your block tower (Step 2). I should've taken a deep breath. I'll help you fix it (Step 3)."

Keep It Going!

1 PLAY GAMES

Play family-friendly games that require keen listening skills, such as Simon Says or Telephone. Family members should feel free to state their needs, including asking others to go slower or repeat something.

SKILLS BEING PRACTICED:

listening and stating needs

2 APOLOGY CARDS

Family members use art supplies to create a card or letter for another person in the family who they've "wronged" in the past. The card should apologize for the mistake that was made. Refer back to Activity 6 for rules on apologizing.

SKILL BEING PRACTICED:

making amends

3 FAMILY MIRROR GAME

Two family members face each other. One person moves their body or face however they like, and the other person has to mirror what they see by copying the movements.

SKILL BEING PRACTICED:

looking at another person's point of view

4 FAMILY TONE PRACTICE

As a family, try saying different statements using first an angry tone, and then a calm one. It's okay to get silly and have fun with this!

SKILL BEING PRACTICED:

tone of voice

HERE ARE SOME STATEMENTS TO GET YOU STARTED:

- "It makes me mad when you do that."
- "I'm sorry for hitting you."
- "That's not fair. We have to take turns."
- "You can't borrow my toys."
- "Please give me some space."

5 FAMILY "I" STATEMENTS

Family members take turns making "I" statements about a feeling they had during the day. Refer back to Activity 2 and follow the template. Example: I felt scared today because another car almost hit me in traffic. I needed to take a deep breath.

SKILLS BEING PRACTICED:

"I" statements, listening, and sharing feelings

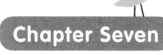

Chapter Seven

Feel Great!

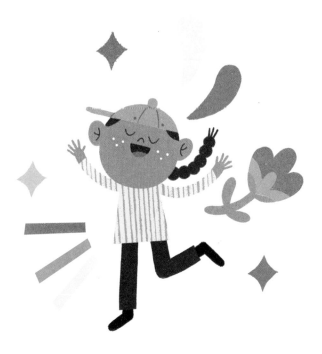

You have worked hard to learn new skills, and now you've made it to the final chapter! The anger management skills in the pages that follow are the same ones you need to feel better all the time. They will help you develop skills that keep your body strong and your mind healthy so you can manage your anger—and feel great, too!

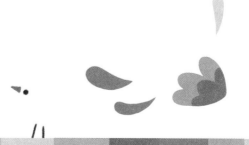

Feed Your Body (and Brain)

The food you eat becomes fuel in your body so that you can run, play, and learn new things. What you may not know is that the food you eat can change your mood, too. Have you ever felt grumpy, and then suddenly felt much better after having a snack? That can happen when you have an empty stomach! Making sure you get enough healthy foods to eat during the day can help you manage your feelings, make your body strong, and keep your brain focused.

What are your favorite healthy foods?
Draw them in the box below:

Find all the healthy foods in the word search:

```
Z  F  F  R  U  I  T  T  P  H
U  S  M  O  O  T  H  I  E  F
T  D  G  T  A  C  C  A  Y  I
D  P  O  P  C  O  R  N  O  E
R  C  H  E  E  S  E  U  G  L
Q  P  M  U  M  Z  Q  Y  U  Z
H  V  E  G  G  I  E  S  R  Q
B  Y  G  C  E  Z  D  D  T  M
M  J  D  A  L  M  O  N  D  S
L  T  P  V  H  U  M  M  U  S
```

Almonds	Veggies	Yogurt
Smoothie	Hummus	Popcorn
Cheese	Fruit	

Rest Your Body (and Brain)

Did you know your brain grows and gets stronger while you sleep? All the things you learn during the day—like math or history (or tools for managing your feelings)—get stored in your brain while you're fast asleep. This means that when you miss out on rest, your brain misses out on its best growing time! Getting enough sleep also puts you in a better mood, which makes it easier to stay in control of your feelings.

For this activity, draw a picture of yourself asleep on the next page. Then read the tips below for getting a good night's sleep. Check off the ones you already do, and circle a new one you'd like to try!

- [ ] Put away screens one hour before bedtime
- [ ] Wear comfy pajamas
- [ ] Don't eat or drink sugary things two hours before bedtime

- [ ] Take a bath or shower
- [ ] Go to bed at the same time every night
- [ ] Read a story
- [ ] Put on lotion
- [ ] Stay in bed all night

Get Active

As you already know, getting exercise helps release angry energy from your body. But even when you feel happy and don't have any anger, physical activity is still great for you. The poem below has lots of ideas for getting exercise, but some of the words are missing! Using the word bank on the next page, fill in the blanks with words that complete the rhyme. When you've completed the poem, under-line the ideas you like best.

Your body needs exercise, and there's lots you can do: You can walk, you can jump, you can kick a ball, too.

You can put on your boots and go for a hike, and other times maybe you'll ride your cool _____.

Other ideas that are good for your heart: swimming or skating or a fun _____.

You can dance to some music and shake your hips, you can take gymnastics and learn back _____.

Throw a Frisbee, play tag, lead your dog on a chase, or challenge your neighbors to a fast running _____.

Before you work out, give your limbs a good stretch, then grab your family and play some _____!

WORD BANK:

Flips   Catch

Race   Bike

Martial art

Stay Away from the Screens!

Screen time is lots of fun. But just like a person can eat too much candy, a person can also spend too much time playing games and watching shows. Too much screen time can make it harder for you to concentrate and control your actions. It can also make you feel cranky and have a hard time relaxing. Have you ever had a big, angry reaction to your parents cutting off your screen time? That happens when your brain has had too much of it!

Help Skylar avoid the screens so that he can get through the maze. Fun, screen-free activity ideas await him (and you) at the end!

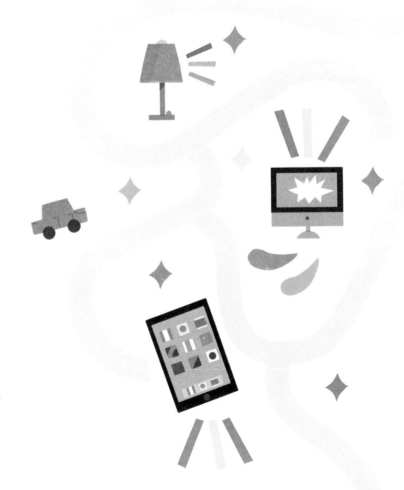

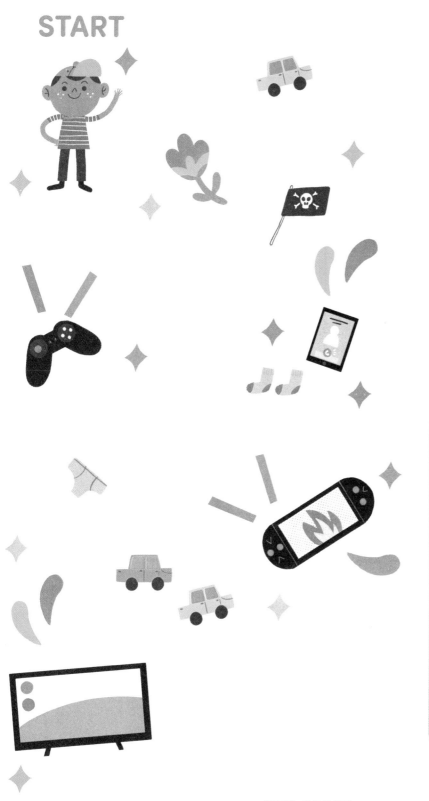

START

END

PUT A STAR NEXT TO YOUR FAVORITE SCREEN-FREE ACTIVITIES:

- ☐ Going outside
- ☐ Playing a card game or board game
- ☐ Reading
- ☐ Drawing or coloring
- ☐ Doing a puzzle
- ☐ Playing with your toys

Self-Care for the Win

In this book, you learned how to take care of your body, your brain, and your feelings. Are you ready to put these skills to the test and see how much you remember? Play the board game on the next page. When you land on a space, answer the question or do the activity. You can play by yourself or with your family.

To play, flip a coin. If you get heads, move one space; if you get tails, move two spaces. (If you have to go back a space and end up on one you've already been on, you don't have to complete it again—but you can if you want!)

START ➡️	Name another word for anger ➡️	What is one way you like to relax? ➡️	MOVE AHEAD ONE SPACE ⬇️
MOVE BACK ONE SPACE ⬇️	Practice taking three slow, deep breaths	Say one thing you're grateful for ⬅️	Name something that makes you mad ⬅️
What's one way that you can get exercise? ➡️	MOVE AHEAD ONE SPACE ➡️	Name something that happens in your body when you get angry ➡️	Name a person you can count on ⬇️
FINISH!! What is something you like about yourself?	Practice a yoga stretch ⬅️	What do you currently see, hear, feel, smell, and taste? ⬅️	MOVE BACK ONE SPACE

Don't Forget to Have Fun!

After going to school, finishing homework, and doing chores, you deserve to have some fun in your day! Hobbies make us feel happier and more patient, which makes us less likely to get annoyed by little things.

Draw a blue circle around the hobbies you do and a red circle around the hobbies you'd like to try.

Cooking and Baking   Gardening

Music   Reading

Biking   Sports

Arts and Crafts   Building

Photography   Painting

Writing   Collecting

Draw a picture of yourself doing your favorite hobby:

Do you have any hobbies that aren't listed
on the previous page? Write them here:

Celebrate Me

Your anger is not the only thing about you, nor is it the most important thing. You're a human being with your own thoughts, feelings, opinions, interests, ideas, and talents. You are worthy and loveable, even when you make mistakes. All of those things about you deserve to be celebrated! Draw a picture of yourself in the frame, and then answer the questions about what makes you, *you!*

Name:

Birthday:

Favorite snacks:

Favorite subject:

What's something you're good at?

What do you want to be when you grow up?

What superpower would you like to have?

Favorite movie:

Favorite color:

Favorite animal:

What is the best part about being you?

Keep It Going!

1 FAMILY FUN TIME

In the previous chapter, you brainstormed free ways to spend time together as a family. Choose one of the ideas from the list to do together. The only rule is that the activity can't involve screens!

SKILLS BEING PRACTICED:

staying away from screens and having fun

2 MAKE A SNACK

As a family, prepare one of the snacks below, and then enjoy it together. Families can also come up with their own snack idea.

SKILLS BEING PRACTICED:

eating healthy, having fun, and staying away from screens

SNACK OPTIONS:
- Trail mix with nuts, dried fruit, peanut butter chips, and M&M's
- Smoothies with fruits and veggies
- Hummus with sliced-up veggies and pita
- Ants on a log (celery with peanut butter and raisins)
- Mini pizzas: pita bread with tomato sauce, mozzarella cheese, and other toppings

3 SCAVENGER HUNT

Go outside and work together as a family to find all the items on the scavenger hunt list below, or come up with your own list. Write down or take a picture of what you find (and leave the items in their places).

> A smooth rock, a pine cone, something yellow, animal tracks, a flower, a squirrel, another kind of animal, a spider web, water (in a creek or pond), an ant hill, something fuzzy, an acorn, two kinds of leaves, a mushroom, something red.

SKILLS BEING PRACTICED:

getting active, having fun, and staying away from screens

4 COLLAGE

Family members use art supplies and old magazines or newspapers to make collages about themselves, their interests, and hopes, then take turns presenting them to each other.

SKILLS BEING PRACTICED:

engaging in hobbies and celebrating strengths

5 FAMILY BOARD GAME

Using Activity 5 as a guide, families create their own board game to practice the problem-solving and self-care skills learned in this workbook.

SKILL BEING PRACTICED:

self-care

Moving Forward

Congratulations—you made it through the entire work-book! You've learned lots of new skills to help you identify your anger, express it safely, solve your problems, and find calm again. That's a lot of new things to learn, and you may forget stuff from time to time. It will help to practice these skills by rereading the activities in the book or asking your parent to run through a skill with you. You may also want to talk about these skills with your friends or other family members—and they may learn something new from you, too!

Once you start using these skills regularly, you'll find that you get in trouble less often and have an easier time getting along better with the people in your life. You'll feel more in control of your feelings and behavior, and you'll feel calmer and happier inside.

I know learning these skills wasn't always easy, so I'm proud of you for sticking with it! I hope that you're proud of yourself, too.

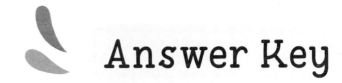

Answer Key

CHAPTER ONE

Activity 1
Decoded words in order: *Grumpy, Furious, Angry, Annoyed, Frustrated*

In ascending order on scale: *Annoyed, Grumpy, Frustrated, Angry, Furious*

CHAPTER TWO

Activity 5
Word search:

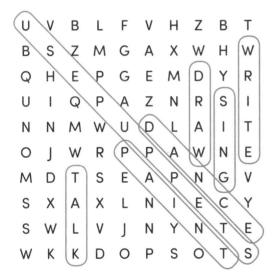

CHAPTER THREE

Activity 1
Riddle: *Breath*
Unscrambled words (top to bottom):
Brain, Think, Feel, Calm
Fill in the blank: *12*
Solve the problem: *Katy is 10 and Blair is 11*

Activity 3

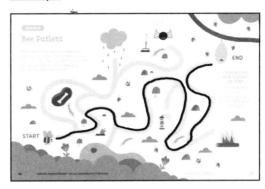

CHAPTER FOUR

Activity 3
Unscrambled words from left to right: *Talk, Cry, Write, Draw, Rip, Yell*

Activity 4
Color-by-number should spell out: *MOVE YOUR BODY*

CHAPTER FIVE

Activity 2
Compromise solutions from top to bottom: *b, a, b*

Activity 3
Decoded words: *Look, Listen, Ask*

Activity 6
Example of finding a solution:

Step 1: Problem that makes you angry

- *When my friend Jarron won't share his video game with me*

Step 2: Brainstorm solutions

- *Grab video game away from Jarron, Tell Jarron I won't play with him unless he lets me use video game, Invite Jarron to my* house but don't share so he knows how it feels, Tell Jarron how I feel when he doesn't share, Shove Jarron, Find other friends to play with who share better

Step 3: Cross out solutions that could hurt people, hurt property, or get me in trouble:

- ~~Grab video game away from Jarron~~, ~~Tell Jarron I won't play with him unless he lets me use video game~~, Invite Jarron to my house but don't share so he knows how it feels, Tell Jarron how I feel when he doesn't share, ~~Shove Jarron~~, Find other friends to play with who share better

Step 4: Talk it over with an adult and cross out any other ideas that might not be realistic or helpful:

- ~~Invite Jarron to my house but don't share with him so he knows how it feels~~, Tell Jarron how I feel when he doesn't share, Find other friends to play with who share better

Step 5: Decide on a solution

- Tell Jarron how I feel when he doesn't share

CHAPTER SIX
Activity 1

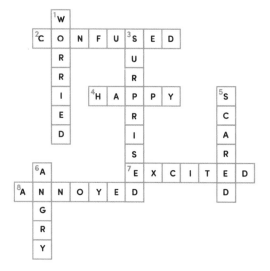

Activity 3
Perspective-taking answers to the scenarios: *a, b, b, a*

Activity 6
Step 1: *Say I'm sorry*
Step 2: *Give a reason why*
Step 3: *Do something kind*

CHAPTER SEVEN
Activity 1
Solved word search:

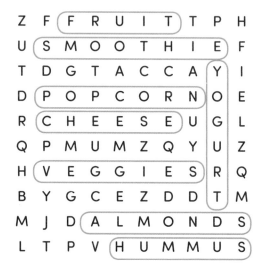

Activity 3
Fill in the blanks in order: *bike, martial art, flips, race, catch*

Activity 4:

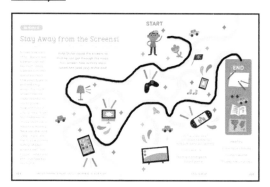

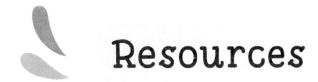

Resources

BOOKS

Positive Discipline by Jane Nelson

This book guides parents on balancing kindness and firmness in their discipline strategies. Parents learn how to bridge communication gaps and reduce power struggles.

The Whole-Brain Child by Daniel Siegel and Tina Payne Bryson

Discusses best practices for responding to children's emotional outbursts and behavioral challenges using current neuroscience.

The Great Behavior Breakdown by Bryan Post

This book covers the most common and challenging behaviors that parents face with their children, and provides insight and strategies for addressing them at home.

APPS

Calm

This app helps children find calm and relaxation using short, guided meditations and peaceful sounds. It also includes "Sleep Stories" for aiding users in falling asleep more easily.

Breathe, Think, Do, with Sesame

More suitable for young children, this app teaches kids how to manage anger and anxiety and find calm.

ORGANIZATIONS

Association for Play Therapy
www.a4pt.org

Visit for more information about play therapy or to find a registered play therapist for your child.

Child Mind Institute
www.childmind.org

Visit for high-quality, research-based articles about children, adolescents, and mental health.

About the Author

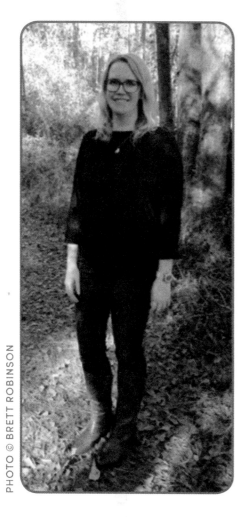

PHOTO © BRETT ROBINSON

AMANDA ROBINSON earned her BA in Psychology from Hardin-Simmons University and her MA in Professional Counseling from Texas State University. She is a licensed professional counselor and registered play therapist. After working at nonprofit agencies for a few years, Amanda is now in private practice, where she works with children and teens with anxiety, anger, and trauma, and also facilitates parenting groups. Amanda is currently the president of her local chapter of the Texas Association for Play Therapy and the secretary of the Austin SandTray Association. She lives in Austin, Texas, and enjoys baking, reading, and hiking.

To learn more about children, mental health, and parenting, visit Amanda's blog at www.amandarobinsonlpc.com/blog